Intermittent Fasting for Beginners

Your Guide to Getting The Most Out Of Your Intermittent Fasting Diet

By
Adam Stephens

Book Description

Do you have Type 2 Diabetes? Are you tired? Are you looking to gain some more energy? Are you trying to shed the excess pounds? If yes, then try intermittent fasting. It is not just a fad, and is gaining popularity. Intermittent fasting (IF) has many mental and health benefits. Losing weight is the most emphasized one, given that obesity and being overweight are the main reasons for experiencing many chronic diseases.

Intermittent Fasting for Beginners is a guidebook that intends to instruct individuals about how to practice IF, what it is, and the diverse methods you can choose from. Moreover, the book also explains the various benefits of intermittent fasting.

Knowing what to eat in a diet is half the battle, which is why Intermittent Fasting for Beginners provides a comprehensive list of food and drinks that you should consume on this diet. Even better, there are several recipes that can be found in this book. Following intermittent fasting patterns won't be difficult. Lastly, there are side effects mentioned so that you can be careful and informed before your decision to undertake IF.

What will you learn in this book?

- What is Intermittent Fasting, or IF?
- Is it safe?
- Methods of IF
- Benefits of IF

- What should you eat?
- Recipes
- Side effects
- Exercise and IF
- And much more!!

Table of Contents

Introduction

Losing weight is difficult, especially when everyone seems to have an opinion on the best techniques to do it. When it comes to weight loss, there is NEVER a "one size fits all" solution. Basic individual differences like sex, age, body type, fundamental medical issues, past experiences with dieting, level of activity, genetics, and even food inclinations can impact an individual's ability to shed weight and maintain it.

Even though there is no perfect diet for weight loss for everyone, there are still certain behaviors that stand true for everyone when it comes to losing weight. These include cutting out soda and sugary drinks, shunning an inactive lifestyle, and concentrating on food quality instead of just on calories.

The following 10 behaviors can support weight loss and also encourage healthy eating:

1.   Monitor where you are starting

Retain a food record for around three days. Write down all the beverages and food you consume and even take note of the portions. Also, recognize the number of times you eat out or buy food in a rush.

2.   Identify your goal and make a plan

Ensure that you are fully aware of what your goal is. Is it to be healthy or to lose weight? How will you attain this goal? Do you plan on cooking more at home from now on? Will you be controlling portions? Make sure that you are specific and have realistic plans by starting small.

3.   Categorize obstacles to your goals and how to overcome them

Is your busy timetable getting in the way of going to the gym? You can try waking up an hour early to workout. Are you always short on the right ingredients? You can find recipes and then go grocery shopping knowing the exact ingredients to purchase.

4.   Classify existing habits that lead to unhealthy eating

Do you unwind and reward yourself by eating junk in front of the TV? Are you skipping lunches often, only to eat excessively later? Do you sometimes over-eat just to finish what's on the plate?

5.   Control your portions

Familiarize yourself and only eat standard serving sizes. For example, are you aware that one serving of pasta is only half a cup?

6. Classify hunger and satiety signals

Be conscious of emotional versus physical hunger. Are you more likely to eat when you are actually hungry, or when you are sad, bored, or anxious? Moreover, you should not completely fill the stomach. Stop eating before getting the "Full" feeling. You might want to consume foods such as legumes, grains, beans, whole grain, and lots of water to help you feel fuller.

7. Concentrate on the positive alterations

Behavior modification takes time. It might take at least three months. Do not give up if you fail a couple of times. You might want to get social support and acknowledge the little changes.

8. Go with the 80/20 rule

Feeling deprived or guilty are the main reasons people cannot stick to healthy eating ways. This is why you must stay on track 80% of the time. However, you should leave some room for a few cheat days.

9. Focus on general health

Bike, walk and dance. You must discover activities you like and do them daily. Rather than sticking to fad diets, opt for fresh, seasonal, whole foods that are high in quality.

10.   Eat slowly and mindfully

Enjoy the whole experience of eating meals. Take the time to enjoy the tastes, aromas, and textures of the food in front of you.

All of these behaviors mentioned above contribute to weight loss; however, one element that everyone tends to forget is TIME. Intermittent fasting is a dietary regimen that focuses on the time that you eat.

The typical reason for trying IF is weight loss. You will be required to fast for a particular period during the day while eating only at specified times. The easier versions of IF do not restrict what you eat, but for effective and quicker weight loss, you might want to cut unhealthy foods as well.

Chapter 1: Intermittent Fasting 101

Intermittent fasting (IF) is a pattern of eating in which an individual will schedule their meals so that they get the most out of them. This diet cycles between periods of fasting and times of unrestricted eating. Intermittent fasting does not always alter what you eat; it regulates *when* you eat.

The idea behind this regimen is to promote change in body composition via loss of weight and fat mass. Moreover, it improves markers of health that are related to ailments, like cholesterol and blood pressure levels.

The roots of this eating pattern are derived from fasting taken up by religious groups, and philosophers Plato and Socrates. When you perform IF, you will have to abstain from all kinds of foods and beverages for approximately 12 hours, up to periods of even a month. This method is preferred over other low-calorie diets because they lead to physiological changes that might cause the body to acclimatize to the calorie restriction and consequently stop additional weight loss.

Intermittent fasting tries to address this issue by cycling amid a low-calorie level for a short time trailed by normal eating that might inhibit these alterations. This eating pattern offers an excellent method of getting lean without having to cut on calories drastically. Additionally, it is a great way to retain muscle mass while getting lean.

Intermittent fasting for weight loss

At its very core, IF basically permits the body to utilize its stockpiled energy by burning off surplus body fat. It is imperative to realize that this is standard, and humans have advanced to fast for smaller time periods – days or hours– without damaging health concerns. Body fat is just food energy that has been deposited. If you do not consume more energy, your body will basically "eat" its own fat for energy. At the end of the day, life is just about balance. The same relates to fasting and eating. Fasting, in spite of everything, is only the flip side of eating. If an individual is not eating, they are fasting.

Here is how intermittent fasting works:

When we consume more and more food, a higher amount of energy is eaten than can be used instantly. Some of this energy is stored away for utilization at a later time. Insulin is the main hormone intertwined in the storing of food energy. As we eat, the insulin level rises, facilitating the storage of excess energy in two distinct ways. Firstly, carbohydrates are broken down into separate glucose (sugar) units that can be interconnected into extensive chains to create glycogen. This is then stockpiled in the muscle.

Nevertheless, there is very minimal storage space for carbs. Once that is used, the liver begins to turn the surplus glucose into fat. This procedure is known as de-novo lipogenesis (meaning "creating new fat").

Some of this freshly made fat is deposited in the liver; however, most of it is distributed to other fat deposits in the body. Though this is a more complex procedure, there is nearly no bound to the quantity of fat that can be produced.

So, two energy-storing balancing systems exist in our bodies. One is effortlessly available; however, with limited storing space (glycogen), and the other is more challenging to access but has virtually limitless storage space (body fat).

The procedure goes in reverse once you start to fast. Insulin levels decrease, cueing the body to begin the burning process of stored energy since additional energy is coming via food. Blood glucose drops, so the body necessitates the procedure of pulling glucose out of the deposits to burn for energy.

The glycogen system is an easily reachable energy source. It is fragmented down into glucose particles to offer energy for the body's other cells. This can deliver enough energy to meet most of the body's requirements for 24-36 hours. Afterward, the body will mainly be cutting down fat for energy.

This way, we can see that the body only stays in two states – the fed condition and the fasting condition. Either we are loading food energy (growing stores), or we are using stored energy (shrinking stores). It is one or the other. When fasting and eating are balanced, then you will see no net change in weight.

If we begin consuming food as soon as we come out of bed till we go back to sleep, then we are basically staying in the fed zone all day. Over time, we might gain weight given that we have not given our body any time to use up the stored food energy.

To reinstate balance or to decrease weight, we might simply have to escalate the amount of time spent consuming food energy. That is how intermittent fasting works

In short, intermittent fasting lets the body consume its deposited energy. The main thing to recognize is that there is nothing wrong with that. This is how our bodies are made. If you are consuming food every three hours, as is generally suggested, then your body will continually utilize the incoming food energy. It might not have to burn a lot of body fat if any. You might just be accumulating fat.

Your body might be storing it for a time when you have nothing to consume. When this transpires, there is an absence of balance; hence you are not indulging in intermittent fasting.

How It Affects Your Cells and Hormones

When you begin fasting, numerous things transpire in your body on the molecular and cellular levels. For instance, your body regulates hormone levels to ensure that stored body fat is more available. Moreover, your cells also initiate imperative repair procedures and alter the expression of genes. Some changes that happen in the body when you begin intermittent fasting include:

Human Growth Hormone (HGH):

When you start to fast, the levels of growth hormone will hit the roof, growing as much as 5-fold. This has advantages for muscle gain and fat loss, to name a few.

Insulin:

Insulin sensitivity increases and the insulin levels drop radically. Lower insulin makes deposited body fat more available.

Cellular repair:

When fasted, your cells will develop enough to engage in cellular repair procedures. This comprises autophagy, a process where cells digest dysfunctional and old proteins that accumulate inside the cell.

Gene expression:

There are alterations in the working of genes associated with longevity and defense against disease.

These modifications in cell function, hormone levels, and gene expression are accountable for the health advantages of intermittent fasting.

Is Intermittent Fasting Safe and Healthy?

Intermittent fasting is known to aid weight loss; however, is it safe to fast for 16 hours?

The truth is intermittent fasting effectively and safely augments weight loss and increases blood sugar. Contrasting from numerous fad diets, IF is supported by ample medical literature. Intermittent fasting is normally effective and safe given it alternates short periods of eating with short periods of fasting. Extending the fasting further than a day can become dangerous since it can put unwarranted stress on the heart.

However, IF can also be unsafe for specific people. Those who have low blood sugar, low blood pressure, or other possibly risky health issues must consult their doctor first.

Individuals who are consuming insulin or other medicines that impact blood sugar might struggle with intermittent fasting because they have to eat more frequently to avoid blood sugar drops. Anybody who has an eating disorder or a past history of eating disorders must avoid intermittent fasting. IF may too closely resemble the cycle of purging or bingeing and activate a relapse in these individuals.

If you are taking medicines that have been consumed with food in the morning or before going to bed, intermittent fasting might not be the best choice; however, there are methods to make it work. Women who are pregnant or want to conceive must take emphasis on eating healthy rather than on weight loss. Remember to check with your doctor first if you are unsure.

Chapter 2: Intermittent Fasting Methods

Suppose a weight loss diet is gaining popularity. It is a process of interchanging cycles of fasting and eating. The best element is that this diet does not limit you on the kinds of foods that can be consumed. Intermittent fasting is all about the timing.

With this diet plan, you will lose weight but also experience several other benefits. It will improve cognitive function, decrease the risk of chronic disease and augment energy levels. It is designed to fast track weight loss goals by dropping calories, crushing stubborn fat, and reforming the metabolism for better performance.

Several techniques are available for incorporating intermittent fasting, all of which are divided into fasting and eating periods. The most common methods of intermittent fasting are:

Intermittent Fasting 16/8

The 16/8 Method incorporates fasting daily for 14–16 hours and limits your everyday eating window to approximately 8–10 hours. During the eating window, you will be able to consume three or more meals. This technique is also called the Lean Gains Protocol. This is a simple method as you can easily stop eating after dinner and skip breakfast.

For instance, if you eat your last meal at 8 p.m. and do not consume anything till mid-day the next day, you are precisely fasting for 16 hours. It is normally suggested that women fast for 14–15 hours, given that they seem to do better with somewhat shorter fasts.

For individuals who get hungry in the morning and prefer consuming breakfast, this technique might be difficult to take up initially. Conversely, many breakfast skippers intuitively eat on this pattern. You can drink coffee, water, and other zero-calorie infusions throughout the fast that can help lessen feelings of hunger.

It is imperative to predominantly eat healthy foods throughout your eating window. This technique will not work if you consume lots of junk food or an unnecessary number of calories. With this method, it is up to you to decide which 16 out of 24 hours you will be fasting. You can opt for an eating window 8 am to 4 pm, noon to 8 pm, 10 am to 6 pm, or any other schedule, as long as it is 16h of uninterrupted non-eating. The best thing is that out of 16h, the chances are that you will be sleeping a minimum of 7-8, so you are actually fasting for 9-8h of fasting every day.

INTERMITTENT FASTING 18/6

Nearly identical to the one 16/8, if you select the 18/6 Intermittent Fasting Schedule, you must fast for 18 hours and eat for only a 6-hour eating window. It is just two more hours of fasting every day, however for a novice faster, these 2 hours can be difficult.

For this reason, we suggest starting with 16/8 for a minimum of a month before moving to 18/6, since you will have a much more pleasurable start with 16/8, which may be the critical difference between quitting and persisting. Slow and steady wins the race – take it gradually and notice the cues given by your body prior to taken up extreme weight loss measures.

Intermittent Fasting 5:2 A.K.A. the Fast Diet

5:2 is a popular method of IF. This version of IF involves limiting your calories to roughly around 500 for two days a week. You will be committing to fast for 2 days, and for the rest of the 5 days, you will sustain a healthy meal regimen. It is vital to focus on high-fiber and high-protein meals to support satiety; nevertheless, it will keep the calories low while fasting.

The idea is that short sessions of fasting keep a person compliant; if you get hungry during a fast day, you only have to wait until tomorrow when you can "slap-up meal" again.

You can select whichever two fasting days (for instance, Wednesdays and Fridays); however, you need to have a non-fasting day between them. Make sure to eat the same quantity of food you usually would on non-fasting days. It is imperative to note that your results will be dependent upon what you eat during the 5 days of non-fasting; therefore, stick to the nourishing and whole diet for maximum results.

Intermittent Fasting 20/4 A.K.A. Warrior Diet

Fitness specialist, Ori Hofmekler, promoted the Warrior Diet. It comprises of consuming small quantities of raw fruits and vegetables during the day and eating one huge meal at night. This method is based on the norm of 'fast-and-feast,' where you can consume small quantities of raw veggies and fruits throughout the day, then eat a big meal in a 4-hour window at night. The 'Warrior Diet' is inspired by the practices of ancient soldiers, who would go fighting or hunting all through the day and concentrate on preparing and eating a night meal only. One drawback that has been noticed with this technique is that it is hard to get all the nutrients the body requires from just one meal.

Individuals following this method will under-eat for 20 hours a day, then devour as much food as they want at night. Throughout the 20-hour fasting time, individuals are allowed to consume small quantities of hard-boiled eggs, dairy products, and raw veggies and fruits, as well as sufficient amounts of non-calorie fluids.

After the 20 hours have passed, individuals can fundamentally binge on any foods they like within a four-hour overindulging window. However, unprocessed, healthy, and organic food choices are encouraged. This diet's food selections are fairly similar to that of the Paleo Diet — typically whole, unrefined foods.

24hr fast A.K.A. Eat Stop Eat

This method entails fasting completely for 24 hours. It can be done once or twice a week. Most individuals start the fast from breakfast and end it at breakfast the next day or even lunch-lunch. Using this technique, you may experience extreme side effects, so it is advised that you should not begin with this method.

In this technique, you will fast from dinner on one day to dinner the next day, amounting to a full 24-hour fast. For instance, if you end your dinner at 7 p.m. Monday, do not consume anything until dinner at 7 p.m. the next day. It can also be done from lunch to lunch or breakfast to breakfast. The end outcome is the same.

Coffee, water, and other zero-calorie drinks can be consumed during the fast; however, no solid foods are allowed. If you are doing this to manage weight, it is imperative that you consume normal or low-calorie meals all through the eating periods. In short, you must eat the same quantity of the food as if you had not been fasting at all.

The possible downside of this technique is that a complete 24-hour fast might be fairly problematic for many individuals. However, you do not have to go all-in right away. It is better to begin with 14–16 hours, then increase from there.

Circadian Rhythm Fasting

The Circadian Rhythm Diet, also known as the Sun Cycle Diet, inspires timing your meals with the rise and fall of the sun. Our bodies are designed to follow the Circadian Rhythm, which is an internal clock that operates 24 hours every day. This cycle regulates our energy levels dependent upon the rhythm of night and day. Therefore if you follow Circadian Rhythm fasting, you will permit daylight to choose your hours.

As soon as the sun comes up, the eating window begins, and you begin your fasting when it gets dark. This impacts the dips and surges in cortisol. That is because cortisol has a noteworthy influence on your thyroid hormones that affect the metabolism of the food you consume.

When cortisol increases in the earlier hours, the metabolism is also accelerated, and you efficiently utilize the food you eat as energy. When cortisol levels fall later in the day, the metabolism instantaneously slows down that makes it more probable that your body will store the food you consume as fat.

The only disadvantage of it is that it actually relies on where you live. In some areas, such as northern Norway, the sun does not set for 76 days in a year, and that is a fasting period that is not recommended.

OMAD Fasting – One-Meal-A-Day a.k.a. 23/1

Another famous fasting schedule is known as One-Meal-A-Day (OMAD). It is precisely what it sounds like – you select a time during the day that is the most appropriate for you to consume your one and only meal of the day. This kind of diet is almost like starving. OMAD diet should not be followed without having a proper plan of getting at least 1200 calories while feasting on that one meal.

Therefore if you opt for this 23/1 fasting – ensure that your meal is a hearty and nourishing one. If you are ardent to experience OMAD, then you must follow a proper nutritionist-made plan, or you can carefully research online for meal plans and recipes.

The Master Cleanse: Lemon Juice & Cayenne Pepper Fast

This prevalent fasting practice came around in the 1940s and was developed by the notorious figure Stanley Burroughs. There are numerous celebrities who follow this cleanse, such as Jared Leto, Beyoncé, Angelina Jolie, and Denzel Washington. The Master Cleanse comprises drinking water only, which is mixed with a hint of cayenne pepper and a half-teaspoon of lemon juice. You are required to consume this five to eight times a day, for five to ten days.

While this fast is not suggested for everybody — and it is not a cure-all or intermittent fast — you may consider this idea when producing your own mixture intermittent fast/diet. One hybrid option may be to drink this formulation from 3 pm to 8 am and eat two calorie-limited meals throughout the hours of 8 am to 3 pm.

Chapter 3: Why opt for intermittent fasting/ Benefits

Fasting in intervals during the week or day is becoming popular as a method to shed extra pounds. Studies suggest that it can also be a good technique to extend lifespan and preserve health. Restricting food consumption to a 6- to 8-hour window every day or eating low-calorie foods two days a week might have significant benefits for overall health.

Weight Loss

Most people take up intermittent fasting to shed extra weight. This claim seems to hold up, especially if the weight loss goal is a short-term one. Largely speaking, IF will make you eat fewer meals in a day. Unless you recompense by consuming much more throughout the other meals, you will end up taking in a smaller amount of calories.

Moreover, intermittent fasting improves hormone function to enable weight loss. Higher growth hormone levels, lower insulin levels, and amplified amounts of norepinephrine (noradrenaline) all increase the breakdown of body fat and simplify its utilization for energy.

As a result, short-term fasting will increase your metabolic rate, making you burn a higher number of calories. Intermittent fasting boosts your metabolic rate and decreases the quantity of food you take in. All things considered, intermittent fasting can be an extremely powerful weight loss instrument.

Change in Cell, Gene, and Hormone Function

When you do not eat for some time, numerous changes ensue in the body. For instance, your body initiates significant cellular healing processes and alters hormone levels to make deposited body fat more available. Some modifications that occur are:

- Insulin levels: insulin levels in the blood drop considerably, which enables fat burning
- Human growth hormone: The blood levels of growth hormone might upsurge approximately 5-fold. Higher levels of this hormone enable muscle gain and fat burning and have several other advantages.
- Cellular repair: The body prompts imperative cellular repair procedures, like eradicating waste material from cells.
- Gene expression: There are valuable changes in numerous molecules and genes associated with protection and longevity against disease.

Reduced Blood Pressure

Intermittent fasting might assist in lowering high blood pressure in the short term. Studies suggest that 16:8 can considerably decrease systolic blood pressure. Moreover, research also shows that the reduction in blood pressure is far more compared to other diets. Sustaining healthy blood pressure is crucial — unhealthy levels can increase your risk for stroke, heart disease, and kidney disease.

However, the research so far indicates that these blood pressure advantages last only while intermittent fasting is practiced. After the diet is over and individuals return to their normal eating pattern, the blood pressure readings also go back to the initial levels.

Reduced Insulin Resistance

Type-2 diabetes is becoming incredibly prevalent in recent decades. Its primary feature is high blood sugar levels in the presence of insulin resistance. Any element that decreases insulin resistance must aid lower blood sugar levels and defend against type-2 diabetes. Interestingly, intermittent fasting seems to help in stabilizing blood sugar levels in individuals with diabetes, given that it resets insulin. The idea is that restricting calories might develop insulin resistance that is an indicator of type-2 diabetes.

Reduced Inflammation and Oxidative Stress

One of the steps towards aging and other chronic disorders is oxidative stress. It involves unbalanced molecules, known as free radicals, which react with other important molecules (such as DNA and protein) and injure them. Numerous studies demonstrate that intermittent fasting might improve the body's resistance to oxidative stress. Moreover, studies also indicate that IF can defend against inflammation, which also leads to many diseases and disorders.

Intermittent Fasting May Help Prevent Cancer

Cancer is a terrible disease categorized by unrestrained cell growth. Fasting has been shown to have numerous beneficial impacts on metabolism that might result in a reduced risk of cancer. Even though human studies and experiments are needed, promising data from animal studies specify that intermittent fasting might aid in preventing cancer.

There is also some proof from human cancer patients, displaying that intermittent fasting decreased some side effects of chemotherapy. Other studies also showed that alternate-day IF might decrease cancer risk by lessening the growth of lymphoma, restraining tumor existence, and decelerating the spread of cancer cells.

Lower Risk of Cardiovascular Issues

Heart disease is presently the world's largest killer. It is recognized that numerous health markers are risk factors linked with either a decreased or increased risk of heart disease. Intermittent fasting has been publicized to enhance several risk factors, including total and LDL cholesterol, blood pressure, blood triglycerides, inflammatory markers, and blood sugar levels. Moreover, with a decrease in insulin level, the risk of many cardiovascular problems also decreases, including congestive heart failure.

Induction of Various Cellular Repair Processes

When an individual takes up intermittent fasting, the cells in the body initiate a cellular "waste removal" process, which is known as autophagy. Autophagy is "a significant detoxification task in the body that cleans out damaged cells." It includes the breakdown of cells and metabolizing broken and dysfunctional proteins that accumulate in cells over time. Increased autophagy might offer protection from numerous diseases, such as cancer and Alzheimer's disease.

Put in a different way, a break from eating allows the body some time to restore and dispose of the junk within the cells that can quicken aging. Food restriction is a recognized way to upsurge neuronal autophagy, which might offer defensive benefits for the brain.

Intermittent Fasting is Good For Your Brain

What is good for the body is usually good for the brain as well. In this regard, intermittent fasting enhances a variety of metabolic features that seem to be important for your brain's health. It includes reduced oxidative stress, decreased inflammation, and a drop in blood sugar levels and insulin resistance.

Numerous studies in rats have demonstrated that IF might increase the progression of new nerve cells, which influence brain function. It also increases levels of a brain hormone known as the brain-derived neurotrophic factor (BDNF). A lack of BDNF has been associated with the occurrence of depression and many other cognitive disorders. Intermittent fasting is also linked with protection from damage from strokes.

Might Help Avert Alzheimer's Disease

Alzheimer's disease is a highly prevalent neurodegenerative disease found around the globe. There is no cure accessible for Alzheimer's, so preventing it from developing in the first place is crucial. An experiment on rats displays that intermittent fasting might delay the inception of Alzheimer's disease or decrease its severity.

It has been shown that a lifestyle that incorporates everyday short-term fasts may considerably improve Alzheimer's symptoms in 9 out of 10 patients, though more human studies need to be conducted for further proof.

May Lengthen Your Lifespan, Helping You Live Longer

One of the most exhilarating applications of IF might be its capability to prolong lifespan. Research on rats has exposed that intermittent fasting lengthens lifespan in the same way as constant calorie constraint. Moreover, intermittent fasting is becoming very prevalent amongst the anti-aging crowd. Given the identified benefits for metabolism and all kinds of health signs, it makes sense that IF could aid you in living a longer and healthier life.

Lower Cholesterol

A variety of studies show that alternate-day fasting might help lower total cholesterol and LDL cholesterol when performed in combination with endurance exercise. LDL cholesterol is the "bad" cholesterol that can increase your danger of stroke or heart disease. It is also observed that intermittent fasting decreases the levels of triglycerides, which are fats contained in the blood that can contribute to heart attack, stroke, or heart disease.

Chapter 4: Who Should Be Careful Or Avoid It?

For some individuals, intermittent fasting is a total game-changer. It is the best strategy to achieve everything ranging from your weight loss goals, to increased mental clarity, to increased energy. However, just because IF is the go-to regimen for some individuals, does not mean it is for everybody.

While intermittent fasting is a great choice for some, for others, it can be hazardous. So who should avoid intermittent fasting? What are the problems that can ensue? And are there any alternatives for individuals who are unable to follow this lifestyle but are still looking for similar advantages?

Insulin-Dependent Diabetics

People who are suffering from Type-1 or insulin-dependent diabetes are one population who can be at a great risk if they follow IF. Given intermittent fasting cycles amid eating and fasting periods, people with diabetes will not be able to retain the insulin levels. It is especially true for individuals who consume anti-diabetic medications.

These medications, precisely insulin, will keep having an impact on blood sugar levels during the fasting periods. It can lead the sugar levels to drop so much that they come to a dangerous level. Diabetics have to uphold stable blood sugar levels to stay fit (via exercise and diet). This can be almost unmanageable with intermittent fasting.

Endurance Athletes

Keeping fit for a marathon or a future Ironman? If so, perhaps intermittent fasting is not for you. Nutrient timing is tremendously significant for sports performance and will be a challenge while taking up an intermittent fasting diet. Endurance sports necessitate increased caloric requirements because of the surplus calories burned.

The effect that endurance exercise has on nutrient requirements before, during, and after an event or long training shift requires constant calorie intake and sufficient macronutrient consumption to restore muscle, restock glycogen stores, and preserve electrolyte balance. Intermittent fasting does not give you a stable dosage of nutrients and calories you need to train, achieve, and recuperate. So, if you have an endurance event forthcoming, you must plan to circumvent intermittent fasting.

People with a History of Disordered Eating

If you are recuperating from a disordered eating condition, intermittent fasting is just not for you.

IF necessitates periods of limitation followed by times of eating bigger meals. This can elicit a dangerous response in people who struggle with confining, binging, or other disordered eating arrangements. In these cases, it is better to circumvent intermittent fasting altogether and follow a more reliable nutrition plan.

Pregnant Women

When you are carrying a baby, you are required to follow a pregnancy-eating regimen that is packed with nutrients and calories to ensure that you and your baby are healthy. Regrettably, you will not get that with intermittent fasting. Individuals with chronic conditions, like diabetes or cancer, will not want to take up intermittent fasting given that it can potentially lead to low blood sugar, insufficient calorie intake, and the likelihood of not meeting acceptable nutrient requirements.

Similarly, the rule applies to women who are expecting and breastfeeding given the increased calorie and nutrient needs. If you are pregnant, you have to eat frequently and in adequate amounts to maintain your and your baby's health. The arrangement of intermittent fasting simply does not permit that.

You have sleep problems

Getting adequate sleep every night is vital for healing and mending muscles from exercise, backing up brain function, and even sustaining emotional well being. When you go to bed hungry, it can become a challenge for the body to unwind and fall asleep, as it will make your brain alert. Consequently, your body feels fidgety. Moreover, insufficient sleep brings numerous health risks, and sleep is when your body does a lot of healing. When you do not eat for a couple of hours, the level of blood sugar will naturally decline, which will wake you up abruptly in the middle of the night.

Disruptions throughout sleep can be damaging to your health, particularly when they occur during the most crucial stage of sleep, called the REM cycle, which helps you retain memory. Not having ample sleep can result in health complications and might hamper memory. Little sleep can actually make you gain weight, as well.

Digestion issues

Having to deal with digestive issues can be cumbersome. If you add an unreliable eating schedule into the mix, it will only lead to more gastrointestinal distress. When you are suffering from issues such as IBS, intermittent fasting will just deteriorate the condition. Periods of prolonged fasting will interrupt the normal actions of the digestive system, resulting in indigestion, constipation, indigestion, and bloating.

You are on medication that has been taken with food

There are some medicines that need to be taken while consuming food, given that they will make you feel light-headed or nauseated without it, amongst other side effects. Intermittent fasting periods can even impact individuals who take several vitamins or supplements each day.

For instance, those who have a low iron sum in their blood or who have anemia might have to take a regular iron supplement to assist in restoring and maintaining iron levels. When you ingest iron supplements with food, it will suppress the nauseating feeling. You must avoid IF when you have to consume a medication that HAS to be taken at an exact time of day and with food.

Intense focus and concentration

Food delivers energy and sustenance, and it empowers you to focus. When you are exceptionally hungry, all you will be able to think about is food. It will divert your attention away from instantaneous tasks.

Even though you might get the hang of this eating regimen eventually, it has a likelihood of hindering your concentration. It is also possible to experience low energy levels and increased fatigue when you fast for longer periods. If you have the kind of job or engage in undertakings where concentration and energy are required, intermittent fasting might not be right for you.

Weak immune system or cancer

Those who have lately experienced a major ailment or are presently facing one must not participate in IF without consulting it with their doctor first. This is because, in the majority of the cases, a sufficient quantity of caloric intake is desirable in order to uphold lean body mass and strong immunity.

For people who suffered from cancer or have weakened immunity, IF is just not workable. Rather you can add other healthy habits that will not only manage your weight but also make you healthy.

People who should avoid IF do not have to be disappointed. You can take up several other healthy habits, such as eating proper meals that are packed with nutrition rather than empty calories. Having water and exercising has many benefits as well.

Chapter 5: What to Eat During Intermittent Fasting

There are no restrictions or specifications regarding the kind of food you can eat or even the amount of food when practicing intermittent fasting. However, the key to successful IF is a well-balanced diet rather than having Big Macs. You should try having nutrient-dense foods like fruits, veggies, whole grains, nuts, beans, and lean proteins.

Water

Even though water isn't technically food, it is imperative if you want to effectively participate in intermittent fasting. Water is a central element for health improvement. One way to check whether you have enough water is to check the color of your urine. It should be pale yellow. If the color is dark yellow, then you are suffering from dehydration that can result in headaches and fatigue. If the thought of plain water does not motivate you, add a few mint leaves, a little bit of lemon juice, or some cucumber slices to your water.

Herbs and spices

Spices and condiments generally have added sugars. So you should be careful of these. Otherwise, you can utilize herbs and spices on an intermittent diet. It is better to choose sea salt or

Himalayan pink salt as a substitute for normal salt because salt tends to cause bloating and swelling in the body. Apple cider vinegar, cocoa powder, Ceylon cinnamon, ginger, rosemary, cilantro, oregano, parsley, turmeric, sea salt, thyme, vanilla bean, and mustard can be consumed on a regular basis.

Avocado

It might seem counterintuitive to consume the highest-calorie fruit when attempting to lose weight. However, due to its high unsaturated fat content, avocados will keep you content in fasting periods—unsaturated fats aid in keeping the body feeling full, which saves you from going into emergency starvation mode.

Fish and seafood

There is a reason 4 ounces of fish in a week is added in the Dietary Guidelines for Americans. It is rich in healthy fats, protein and contains sufficient amounts of vitamin D.

Nuts, Seeds

Nuts and seeds can be used in moderate quantities to create some incredible textures. The best technique is to roast these seeds and nuts because this removes anti-nutrients. Normally raw nuts can be added to give flavor to meals. You may also eat them as snacks, because they have healthy fats. You may eat cashews, raw almonds, hazelnuts, pecans, macadamia nuts, and walnuts; almond flour, coconut flour; tiger nut flour occasionally.

Hummus

One of the tastiest and creamiest dips is hummus and is an excellent plant-based protein. It offers the best solution for boosting the nutritional content of popular foods such as sandwiches—merely sub it in for mayo. If you are daring enough to make your own hummus, do not forget that the hidden ingredients to an impeccable recipe are garlic and Tahini.

Cruciferous veggies

Foods such as Brussels sprouts, broccoli, and cauliflower are packed with the f-word — fiber! When you are eating through some intervals, it is imperative to consume fiber-rich foods that will keep you steady and aid your poop factory to run effortlessly. Fiber is also known for helping you feel full, which might be a good thing if you cannot eat for 16 hours. Cruciferous veggies can also reduce your cancer risk.

Potatoes

This is to prove that not all white foods are bad. Studies from the '90s discovered that potatoes were one of the most gratifying foods. Another research from 2012 exposed that consuming potatoes as part of a healthy diet can aid in losing weight. However, it is the way you consume it that matters. Naturally, having a bucket of French fries will give you the opposite result.

Beans and legumes

Your favorite addition to chili might be a good companion to the intermittent fasting lifestyle: food, especially carbs, delivers energy to your body. We are not advising you to carb-load to ludicrous levels; however, it certainly would not hurt to add some low-calorie carbohydrates such as legumes and beans into your eating strategy. It can keep you active throughout your fasting hours. In addition, items such as chickpeas, peas, black beans, and lentils have been shown to reduce body weight, even without calorie limitations.

Probiotics

You know what the little critters in your gut like the most? - Uniformity and variety. That implies that they are not content when they are hungry. And when your gut is not pleased, you might experience some exasperating side effects, such as constipation. To offset this distastefulness, add probiotic-rich foods such as kombucha, kefir, and sauerkraut into your diet.

Berries

Berries are packed with crucial nutrients. And that is not even the best part. According to a study that was conducted in 2016, people who consumed a whole cluster of flavonoids, like those conveyed in strawberries and blueberries had smaller increases in BMI over a 14-year era than individuals who did not consume berries.

Eggs

One big egg offers 6.24 grams of protein and is prepared within minutes. Remember that consuming a lot of protein is important for keeping you full and developing muscle, particularly when you are consuming less food.

In a 2010 study, it was discovered that men who ate eggs rather than a bagel were slightly less hungry and ate less during the day. In short, when you are searching for something to eat during your fasting period, you can get out some eggs to boil. You can then consume the hard-boiled eggs when the time is right.

Whole grains

Eating carbs and being on a diet might seem like they fit in two diverse buckets. You will be super pleased to know that this is not ALWAYS the case. Whole grains deliver lots of protein and fiber, so consuming a little will go a long way to keeping you full. So go out of your comfort zone to enjoy a whole-grain paradise of bulgur, farro, Kamut, millet, amaranth, sorghum, or freekeh.

Chapter 6: Recipes

Even though intermittent fasting does not restrict you on the kind of food you consume or the quantity, if your goal is to lose weight, try to limit your meals to low-calorie foods. Attempt to avoid junk food or fast food at all costs; since it defeats the purpose. Throughout your eating window, do not binge; otherwise, you might just end up gaining weight. You might also want to incorporate Keto or Paleo recipes as they are low in calories and aim at shedding the extra weight.

Paillard of chicken with lemon & herbs

Ingredients

- 6 skinless chicken breasts
- 2 tbsp olive oil
- ½ tbsp balsamic vinegar
- 140g-bag rocket
- 25g parmesan
- Lemon wedges

For the marinade

- 2 garlic cloves
- 3 rosemary sprigs, leaves finely chopped
- 6 sage leaves, finely shredded

- Zest 1 lemon and juice of ½
- 3 tbsp olive oil

Directions

Place each piece of chicken breast amid 2 sheets of parchment paper or cling. Using a rolling pin, bash on both sides to flatten the chicken to form an even layer approximately 0.5cm thick. Put it in a dish.

To prepare the marinade, crush the garlic and add a pinch of salt utilizing a pounder. Put in the sage and rosemary, and give all the ingredients a good hammering. Stir the lemon juice and zest, ground black pepper, and olive oil.

Pour the dressing onto the chicken, guaranteeing that it is well coated—cover and chill for a minimum of 2 hrs. Warm up the barbeque. After the flames die down, spread the coals and cook the chicken for 1-2 minutes on both sides.

Put it on a board and leave to cool for a few minutes. In the meantime, pour the balsamic vinegar and oil into a large bowl. Add the rocket and some seasoning. Mix together, and then add some Parmesan shaving over it. Serve this salad with chicken and lemon to squeeze over.

Easy Jerk Chicken Drumsticks

Ingredients

- 2 pounds chicken drumsticks or thighs
- 2 Scotch bonnet peppers, stemmed and seeded
- 3 tbsp lime juice
- 4 scallions, chopped plus extra to serve
- 4 garlic cloves
- 2 bay leaves
- 3 tbsp fresh thyme leaves or 1 tbsp dried thyme
- 1-inch fresh ginger root, peeled and chopped
- 1 tbsp honey
- 1 ½ tsp salt
- 1 tbsp black peppercorns
- 2 tsp allspice berries
- ½ tsp ground cinnamon
- ½ tsp smoked paprika

Directions

Using a small knife, pierce the chicken all over. Take a blender and place the garlic, scallion, bay leaves, lime juice, Scotch bonnet peppers, thyme, honey, salt, black peppercorns, allspice berries, smoked paprika, and cinnamon. Blend them together until it is smooth. Toss the jerk seasoning with the chicken drumsticks—cover and chill for at least 1 hour (or even till 1 day).

Next, preheat the oven to 400°F. Line a baking tray with foil and casually grease with olive oil.

Then bake the chicken for 40-45 minutes or till cooked through. Remove from the oven, sprinkle with chopped scallion and serve.

Low Carb Burgers

Ingredients

- 1 lb ground beef
- 1 tsp hot smoked paprika
- 2-3 garlic cloves, minced
- 1 ½ tsp dried oregano
- 1 tbsp olive oil
- Salt and black pepper to taste

Directions

Take a big bowl and put the ground beef, garlic, smoked paprika, and oregano—season with salt and pepper to taste. Combine properly and create four 1-inch thick patties. Place them on a tray and let it cool for 5 minutes.

Heat around 1 tablespoon of olive oil and place the patties in the pan. Next, cook for 3-5 minutes on each side, or until they are cooked to your preferred doneness. Serve with your favorite condiments and buns such as pickles, crisp bacon, paleo mayo, lettuce, onion, etc.

Steak with Scallion-Ginger Sauce

Ingredients

- 2 10-oz. 3/4-inch-thick boneless strip steaks
- 1/4 teaspoon kosher salt
- 4 teaspoons canola oil
- 2 scallions, thinly sliced
- 1/4 teaspoon black pepper
- 2 teaspoons minced fresh ginger
- 1 clove garlic, minced
- 1/4 cup dry sherry
- 2 tablespoons low-sodium chicken broth
- 2 teaspoons oyster sauce
- 1 tablespoon unsalted butter
- 2 teaspoons sesame seeds

Directions

Warm a 12-inch pan at medium heat while seasoning the steaks with pepper and salt. In the pan, swirl 2 tsp oil.

Add steaks and cook till it is brown on one side, which takes around 3 to 4 minutes.

Turn the side and cook for another 3-4 minutes.

Transfer it to a plate and cover it with foil. Add the rest of the 2 tsp oil, white and light green scallion and ginger to pan; sauté for one minute. Next, put garlic and sauté for 30 seconds. Then add broth and sherry.

Stir and cook till the liquid reduces by half. Mix in oyster sauce. Take away the skillet from heat; add butter and whirl until the sauce is creamy. Cut steaks; spoon sauce on it. Top with scallion greens and sesame seeds.

Spinach-Mozzarella Stuffed Burgers

Ingredients

Makes 4 patties

- 1½ lbs ground chuck
- 1 teaspoon salt
- ¾ teaspoon ground black pepper
- 2 cups fresh spinach, firmly packed
- ½ cup shredded mozzarella cheese (about 4 oz)
- 2 tablespoons grated Parmesan cheese

Instructions

Take a medium bowl and combine pepper, salt, and ground beef. Scoop around ⅓ cup of blend and with dampened hands make 8 patties roughly ½-inch thick. Let them refrigerate.

Next, place spinach in the pan at medium heat—Cook for 2 minutes. Drain and let the beef cool. Using your hands, squeeze the spinach to remove all the liquid.

Next, chop the spinach, and place it in a separate bowl. Then stir in mozzarella cheese and Parmesan. Take out roughly ¼ cup of filling and mound in the middle of 4 patties.

Cover with the rest of the 4 patties, and cover the edges by pressing them together. Take each of these patties in your hand and cup it to even out the edges. Press from the top so that the patty flattens slightly into a single thick one.

Next, heat the grill or a pan to medium-high. Grill the burgers for around 5 to 6 minutes on every side. Serve for a delicious meal!

Harissa Chickpea Stew with Eggplant and Millet

Ingredients

- 1 cup millet
- Kosher salt

- 2 tablespoons ghee
- 1 large Japanese eggplant
- Freshly ground black pepper
- 1 onion, diced
- 3 garlic cloves, minced
- 1 fourteen-ounce can of pureed tomatoes
- 1 fourteen-ounce can chickpeas, drained
- 2 tablespoons Harissa paste
- Garnish: 1 bunch cilantro

Directions

Take 2 cups of water and fill it in a medium saucepan. Then add a pinch of salt and millet. Let it boil by covering and cooking for approximately 25 minutes. After the millet is cooked, remove the lid, botch with a fork and let it cool.

In the meantime, heat 1 tablespoon of oil or ghee in a skillet over medium heat. Put the eggplant and season it with pepper and salt. Keep cooking until it is golden brown, and keep adding more oil if required so that the eggplant does not stick to the skillet.

This will take around 10 minutes. Transfer the eggplant to a bowl and let it cool.

Add the rest of 1-tablespoon oil or ghee to the skillet, and after placing the onions, cook until it is golden brown. Then put the garlic and cook for around two more minutes. You can season it with pepper and salt.

Next, you need to add chickpeas, tomatoes, and the Harissa. Then add the eggplant to the same skillet and reduce the heat. Let it simmer for 15 minutes. Divide the millet into two bowls and add the stew above it. Serve warm after garnishing with cilantro.

Salmon Burgers with Mustard Sauce

Ingredients

- 12 oz. salmon fillets, skin removed and finely chopped
- 1 egg, beaten
- 3 cloves garlic, minced
- 3 green onions, chopped
- 1 tbsp Paleo Hoisin sauce
- 1/2 tsp salt
- 1/4 tsp pepper
- Dash of cayenne
- 1/4 cup almond flour
- Coconut oil for the pan

For the mustard sauce

- 1/4 cup mayonnaise
- 3 tbsp spicy Paleo mustard

- 1-2 tbsp lemon juice

Directions

Take a large bowl, and mix all of the ingredients properly. Using your hands, form 4-5 burger patties, packing them firmly. In a different bowl, stir the ingredients for the mustard sauce.

You can add the lemon juice according to your taste. Then set it aside. Melt around a tablespoon of coconut oil in a pan and place the salmon patties.

Cook for 4-6 minutes on each side until browned throughout. Serve warm, trickled with mustard sauce.

Thai prawns with pineapple & green beans

Ingredients

- 1 tbsp vegetable oil
- 2 lemongrass stalks, tough outer leaves removed, the rest finely chopped
- 1 thumb-sized piece ginger, shredded
- 100g fresh pineapple chunks
- 100g green bean
- 100g whole cherry tomato
- 200g raw king prawn
- 1 small pack Thai basil leaves or regular basil leaves

For the sauce

- 4 tbsp lime juice, plus wedges to serve
- 2 tbsp liquid chicken stock
- 1 tbsp fish sauce
- 1 tbsp soft brown sugar

Directions

Mix the ingredients of the sauce in a bowl and set it aside. Then heat up the oil, taking a big wok. Heat the oil in a large wok. Next, sauté the ginger and lemongrass until it is golden brown. Mix in the pineapple, cherry tomatoes, and beans.

Then stir-fry for 3-5 minutes until the beans are cooked. Add the prawns and the sauce. Stir-fry for another 3-5 minutes until the prawns are prepared and roasted, then throw in the basil leaves. Serve with lime, and the residual basil leaves speckled over.

Slow Cooker Beef and Cabbage Stew

Ingredients

- 1 medium head of cabbage, sliced
- 2 pounds chuck roast,
- 6 medium carrots,
- 1 medium onion, chopped

- 2 garlic cloves, minced
- 2 medium tomatoes, chopped
- 1 tsp salt
- ½ tsp black pepper
- 1 tsp paprika
- ½ tsp chili flakes
- 1 tbsp homemade pickling spice
- 2 cups beef stock or water
- 2 tbsp chopped fresh parsley

Directions

Take a slow cooker and add onions, beef cubes, garlic, and carrots. Top it with sliced cabbage, parsley, and tomato. Using a small bowl, mix the beef soup, pepper, salt, paprika, chili flakes, and pickling spice.

Pour over the vegetables and meat. Cover the cooker and cook it for around 6-8 hours on low heat. Remove the lid, mix, and add salt to taste. Garnish with chopped parsley and serve.

Bacon Asparagus Mini Frittatas

This mini frittata recipe makes the perfect breakfast. They're filling, nutritious, and delicious.

Ingredients

- 1 cup chopped asparagus (approx. 7–8 spears)
- 4 slices bacon, diced
- 2 Tablespoons chopped onions
- 8 eggs, whisked
- 1/2 cup (120 ml) coconut milk (from a can)
- Salt and pepper to taste

Directions

Preheat the oven to 350 F or 175 C. Then, take a large bowl and put all the ingredients together. If you prefer a crispier texture, then you might want to cook the bacon before.

Ensure that the asparagus is chopped into tiny pieces, which will make it easier to prepare in the oven. Secondly, whisk all the ingredients together in the mixing bowl. Next, you need to fill a muffin pan with this mixture.

Try to ensure the mixture is equally spread so that there are the same amounts of bacon and asparagus in all muffins. You should utilize a silicone muffin pan or muffin liners to avoid the muffins from sticking.

Lastly, bake for approximately 25-30 minutes in the oven. Check the muffin by poking a stick in the middle. If it's not gooey, then you it's done.

Creamy Tuscan Garlic Chicken

This delicious dish comes with an interesting creamy garlic sauce mixed with sun-dried tomatoes and spinach. You can prepare this restaurant-quality meal in 30 minutes.

Ingredients

- 1½ pounds boneless skinless chicken breasts sliced thinly
- 1 cup heavy cream
- 1/2 cup sun-dried tomatoes
- 1/2 cup chicken broth
- 1 teaspoon garlic powder
- 1 teaspoon Italian seasoning
- 1/2 cup parmesan cheese
- 2 Tablespoons olive oil
- 1 cup spinach chopped

Instructions

In a big pan, add olive oil and cook the chicken on medium-high heat for 3-5 minutes until it is brown on both sides. Make sure that it is not pink from the center. Move the chicken from the pan and set it aside.

Next, you need to add the chicken broth, heavy cream, Italian seasoning, garlic powder, and Parmesan cheese. Whisk it on medium to high heat till it begins to thicken. Add the sundried tomatoes and spinach. Let the mix simmer till the spinach begins to wilt. Add the chicken back to the pan and serve over pasta if desired.

Cheesy Brussels sprouts

Who says you can't have cheese while you are on a diet?

Ingredients

- 3-4 tablespoons extra virgin olive oil
- 2 pounds Brussels sprouts, halved or quartered depending on size
- 4-6 ounces bacon, cut into 1/4-inch pieces
- 1 cup diced onion
- 2 cups heavy cream
- 1/2 teaspoon kosher salt
- 1/2 cup sour cream
- 8 ounces grated smoked Gouda cheese
- 8 ounces grated, part-skim mozzarella cheese
- 4 ounces crumbled feta cheese for garnish
- 1 teaspoon garlic salt
- Black pepper

Directions

In a large, yet shallow skillet, take around 3-4 tablespoons of olive oil and heat it. After the oil is hot, cautiously place the

Brussels sprouts into the pan. Do not stir initially. Cook the sprouts for approximately 15 minutes, rarely mixing, so the sprouts burn on at least a couple of sides. Remove the sprouts from the pan and set them aside.

Put the bacon in the pan; sauté for around 5 minutes. Stir till the bacon is crispy. Remove bacon onto a paper towel-lined plate and put it aside. Bring the heat to medium. Next, take the bacon fat and add onion to it. Stir-fry for 5 minutes till the onions have caramelized a little.

Then you need to add sour cream, heavy cream, mozzarella, Gouda, and feta; mix well. Decrease the heat to medium-low after the cheese melts. Put the Brussels sprouts back in the pan with the cheese sauce and mix it up. If the sauce comes out to be very thick, you can add a little heavy cream to it. To make it even more delicious, season it with pepper and garlic salt. Serve right after you garnish with reserved bacon.

Vegetarian Lettuce Wraps

Ingredients

- 3 tablespoons Hoisin sauce
- 3 tablespoons reduced-sodium soy sauce
- 2 tablespoons rice vinegar
- 1 teaspoon sesame oil
- 2 teaspoons canola oil — or grapeseed oil

- 1 package extra-firm tofu — (12- to 14-ounces),
- 8 ounces baby Bella cremini mushrooms
- 1 can water chestnuts — (8 ounces), finely chopped
- 2 cloves garlic — minced
- 2 teaspoons freshly grated ginger
- 1/4 teaspoon red pepper flakes — omit if sensitive to spice
- 4 green onions — thinly sliced,
- 8 large inner leaves romaine lettuce
- Optional for serving: grated carrots

Instructions

Take a small bowl and stir the Hoisin, rice vinegar, soy sauce, and sesame oil. Then set it aside. Press the tofu amid paper towels to squeeze the liquid from it. Get more paper towels and press again. Heat 2 teaspoons of canola oil in a nonstick skillet at medium heat. After the oil is hot, crush in the tofu and let it cook for 5 minutes.

Next, add the diced mushrooms and continue cooking till there is no remaining tofu liquid and it starts to turn golden, which will take around 3 minutes.

Stir in the garlic, water chestnuts, red pepper flakes, ginger, and half of the green onions and cook till fragrant. Pour the sauce over the top of the tofu mixture and stir. Cook for 30-60 seconds. Spoon the tofu mix into lettuce leaves and enjoy it.

Teriyaki Ginger Tuna Skewers

Ingredients

- 15 ounces teriyaki sauce
- 1 tablespoon fresh ginger, minced
- 3 ounces sesame oil
- 1 tablespoon sugar substitute
- 1 teaspoon fresh garlic, minced
- 1 lemon, juiced
- 2 pounds fresh tuna steak, cut into 1-inch cubes
- 1 tablespoon sesame seeds, toasted

Directions

Soak the bamboo skewers in water for around 30 minutes to an hour. Combine the marinade ingredients in a bowl. Submerge tuna cubes in the marinade, then cover it, and put it in the fridge for a minimum of 30 minutes. Then preheat the grill pan at a high temperature.

Remove the tuna from the marinade and skewers from water. Then thread the tuna onto the skewers. Keep the skewers on the grill. Turn the sticks by hand to keep them from burning. This will be done within 3-4 minutes. Before serving, sprinkle with sesame seeds.

Mini chocolate pumpkin pie

Ingredients

- 3 Tablespoons coconut butter (or pumpkin puree)
- 3 Tablespoons cacao powder
- 3 Tablespoons ghee
- 1 teaspoon pumpkin pie spice (a blend of ground cinnamon, nutmeg, ginger, cloves)
- 3 Tablespoons coconut cream
- Sweetener of choice

Directions

Melt the coconut cream, coconut butter, and ghee in a bowl. Put the spices and cacao powder. Mix well and place into the piecrusts. Refrigerate for 1-2 hours for better consistency. Sprinkle the pumpkin pie spice or cacao on top.

Spinach, Goat Cheese & Chorizo Omelet

Ingredients

- 4 ounces chorizo sausage
- 1/2 Tbsp butter
- 4 eggs
- 1 Tbsp water

- 2 ounces crumbled fresh goat cheese
- 2 cups baby spinach leaves
- Sliced avocado (optional)
- 1/4 cup salsa verde (optional)

Directions

Remove chorizo from its cover and fry at medium heat in a sauté pan until it is cooked. In the meantime, whisk the eggs and water in a separate bowl. Next, take the chorizo out from the pan and set it aside.

Wipe the pan off the residual fat using a clean kitchen tissue. Melt the butter in the pan at low heat and add the beaten eggs.

Then place the spinach, Chorizo, and crushed goat cheese in half of the egg blend. Cook at low heat for 3 minutes till lightly firm. Next, fold the empty side over to the other.

Cover the pan with foil and leave at low heat for extra few minutes until the eggs are cooked completely. If the bottom is browning too rapidly, turn off the stove.

Leave the pan covered for another 10 minutes, and the rest of the heat will "bake" it until the center is entirely cooked. Plate it with avocado slices and salsa verde.

Chapter 7: Possible Side Effects

Even though weight loss is a major reason individuals opt for intermittent fasting, there are numerous other health advantages. You might experience decreased inflammation, reduced bloating, improved digestion, amplified mental clarity, better sleep, and even control your sugar cravings. If you are ready to give it a try, then you must be aware of certain side effects. Always remember that your body needs time to familiarize yourself with these extreme changes.

Hunger

When you are used to consuming five to six meals in a day, your body comes to expect food at certain times. Ghrelin, a hormone, is accountable for making you feel hungry. It normally peaks at breakfast, lunch, and dinnertime and is partly controlled by food intake. When you first begin fasting, ghrelin levels will continue to peak at these times, and you will feel the same levels of hunger.

Initially, when you begin intermittent fasting, it is imperative that you have the willpower to continue. The majority of the time, you will have the worst feelings of hunger during days 3 to 5.

It is suggested that you try and keep your belly full by consuming a lot of water, and this is a great technique for the first two weeks to manage hunger. Moreover, it will keep you alert and satiate that routine of having to put something in your mouth throughout the fasting period.

Within 30 minutes of waking up, drink a minimum of 12 ounces. If you sense a pang of hunger, drink an additional 12 ounces or more. One lesson intermittent fasting will show you is that what you believed was hunger was perhaps boredom or thirst.

Headaches

When you indulge in intermittent fasting, your body will initially try and get used to this new eating pattern, and there is a possibility of experiencing dull headaches that come and go. Another factor that contributes to the headache is the lack of water consumption. Dehydration during the fasting or eating window will result in severe headaches. For this reason, you must drink lots of water. If you experience a decrease in blood sugar levels, the chances of getting headaches also increase. Stress hormones released by the brain might also result in headaches. With time, your body will get used to this new eating timetable; however, try to stay as stress-free as possible.

Low Energy

When you start intermittent fasting, your body will no longer receive a constant fuel source that you are used to getting from consuming foods all day long. Expect to feel sluggish in the initial weeks. Attempt to keep your day as stress-free as possible so you can expend the lowest amount of energy possible. You may want to give exercise a brief break. Sleeping more often can also be helpful.

Bathroom Trips

Because you are drinking oceans of water to keep yourself hydrated and give a feeling of being full, you are going to feel the need to run to the bathroom more frequently. It could even be twice in an hour. There is no way around this because it is not advised to reduce your water intake.

Irritability

Feeling hungry is an actual phenomenon, and it sucks. It is expected that when you begin IF, you will experience crankiness. This is mainly due to a decrease in your blood sugar levels while you have to deal with the other side effects of IF. Just stay away from people who create a fuss or make you feel annoyed.

Heartburn, Bloating, and Constipation

Your stomach forms acid to facilitate the digestion process, so when you are not eating, you might feel heartburn (this side effect is not very common compared to the others). This can range from mild uneasiness to belching all day to full-on pain. Time will treat this side effect, so just continue your water routine, prop yourself up when you sleep, and when you do eat, avoid greasy, peppery foods that can make your heartburn worse. If your heartburn does not go away, please consult your doctor. Intermittent fasting can also lead to constipation if you are not keeping yourself hydrated. This can result in bloating and discomfort.

Cravings

Naturally, when you are prevented from having a particular food, the chances are that you will want it even more badly. During intermittent fasting, you will be going through extended periods of fasting. So chances are, you will only be able to think about foods that you cannot consume. Once cravings kick in, it will get harder to follow the eating pattern. The majority of the time, people crave sweets and/or refined carbs, given that your body is looking for that glucose hit.

Chapter 8: Exercise & Fasting

The success of any exercise program or weight loss plan is contingent upon how safe it is to maintain over time. If your eventual objective is to reduce body fat and sustain your fitness level while doing intermittent fasting, you must stay in the safe region. Here are some specialist tips to aid you in doing just that.

Eat a meal around your moderate- to a high-intensity exercise routine

When it comes to intermittent fasting, the main thing is timing. For this tip especially, you will have to take care of your meal timing. Performing a high to moderate intensity workout right after consuming a big meal is also an issue. So make sure you give ample time between the workout and your meal but not too much that you experience a loss of energy. When you consume a meal, your body will have some glycogen stores to tap into to energy your exercise routine.

Stay hydrated

Intermittent fasting only restricts solids, so there is no limitation on water. Rather it is better to have lots of water while fasting. Staying hydrated will not only decrease the level of fat in the body but also have a positive impact on your skin.

Keep your electrolytes up

If you are looking to keep your electrolytes up, then try out a great source of low-calorie hydration. A good drink can be coconut water. It refills electrolytes, is low in calories, and has a pretty good flavor. Sports drinks and Gatorade are high in sugar, so try to avoid them.

Keep the duration and intensity fairly low

If you work out too hard or exert yourself too much, you will begin to feel dizzy or lightheaded. For this reason, you must take a break. Learn to listen to your body and exercise accordingly.

Consider the kind of fast

If you are indulging in a 24-hour intermittent fast, you must stick to low-intensity exercises like:

- Walking
- Restorative yoga
- Gentle Pilates

However, if you are practicing a 16:8 fast, then the majority of the 16-hour fasting period is sleep, evening, and early in the day, so sticking to a specific kind of exercise is not as dangerous.

Listen to your body

The most imperative advice to be attentive to when exercising while following intermittent fasting is to listen to your body. When exercising, if you start to feel dizzy or weak, the likelihood is that you are experiencing low blood sugar.

Feeling dehydrated might be another reason. In such situations, it is best to choose a carbohydrate-electrolyte drink to consume immediately and then follow up with a balanced meal. Though exercising and intermittent fasting might work for some individuals, others might not feel relaxed doing any kind of exercise while fasting.

Conclusion

Intermittent fasting has been trendy for a while now and is known to show some incredible results. This is especially true for weight loss. It is an eating regimen in which a person will cycle between periods of fasting and eating. The best feature of this eating plan is that it does not restrict you on the kinds of foods that you can consume.

The book offers a brief description as to what intermittent fasting is and the diverse methods. Understanding these methods will help you, as it will allow you to choose a method that works best for you. Pick a method that corresponds to your schedule so that it becomes easy for you to follow the eating regimen.

To convince you, this book explains the numerous benefits of IF so that you can take up this way of eating confidently. You will also be aware of the several possible side effects of this diet. As a result, you will be able to weigh your options easily, which will help you make an informed decision.

The best feature of this guidebook is that it tells you what you can consume in this eating regimen, making your shopping trips a lot easier. Recipes are also provided in this all-inclusive guidebook, which allows you to cook in time so that timings can be followed.

We hope that this book has been informative and given you the tools necessary to succeed with IF.